ALKALINE DIET

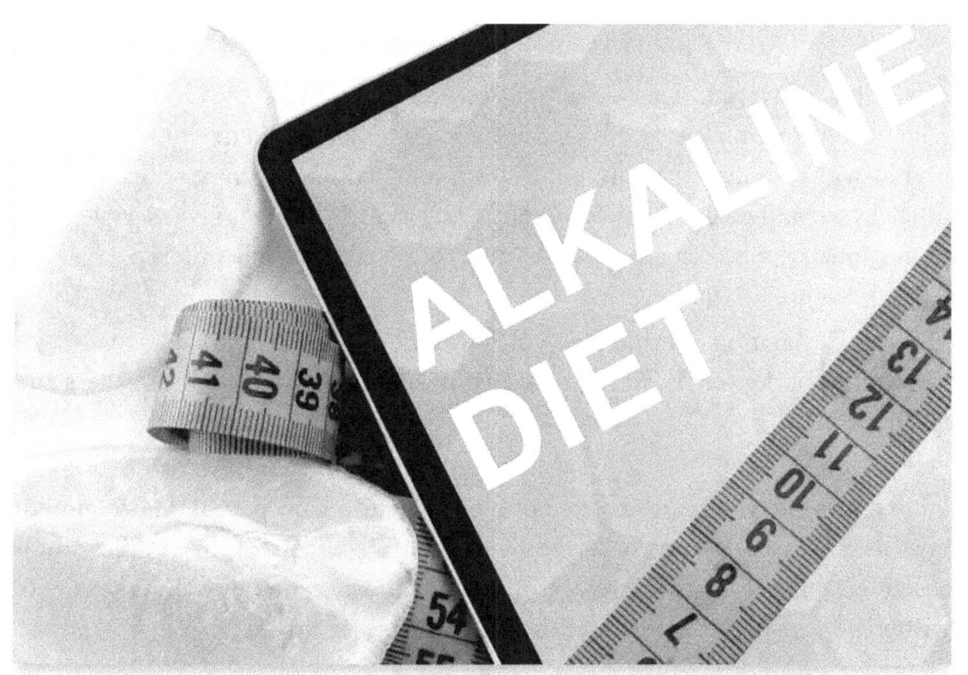

By Julia Bond

Copyright © 2017 by Julia Bond

The trademarks that are used are without any consent, and the publication of the trademark is without permission or backing by the trademark owner. All trademarks and brands within this book are for clarifying purposes only and are the owned by the owners themselves, not affiliated with this document.

Disclaimer and Terms of Use: The Author and Publisher has strived to be as accurate and complete as possible in the creation of this book, notwithstanding the fact that he does not warrant or represent at any time that the contents within are accurate due to the rapidly changing nature of the Internet. While all attempts have been made to verify information provided in this publication, the Author and Publisher assumes no responsibility for errors, omissions, or contrary interpretation of the subject matter herein.

Any perceived slights of specific persons, peoples, or organizations are unintentional. In practical advice books, like anything else in life, there are no guarantees of results. Readers are cautioned to rely on their own judgment about their individual circumstances and act accordingly.

This book is not intended for use as a source of legal, medical, business, accounting or financial advice. All readers are advised to seek services of competent professionals in the legal, medical, business, accounting, and finance fields.

TABLE OF CONTENTS

INTRODUCTION

What if you knew about a weight loss program that would help you lose weight and feel younger? Would you try it? The alkaline diet and lifestyle has been around for over 60 years, yet many people aren't familiar with its natural, safe and proven weight loss properties!

The alkaline diet is not a gimmick or a fad. It's a healthy and easy way to enjoy new levels of health. In this post you'll learn about what this dietary plan is, what makes it different, and how it can produce life-changing results for you, your waistline and your health.

Are you enjoying a slim and sexy body today? If so, you're in the minority.

Sadly, over 65 percent of Americans are either overweight or obese. If you're overweight, you probably experience symptoms of ill-health like fatigue, swelling, sore joints, and a host of other signs of poor health.

Worse yet, you probably feel like giving up on ever enjoying the body you want and deserve. Perhaps you've been told that you're just getting older, but that simply isn't the truth. Don't buy into that lie. Other cultures have healthy, lean seniors who enjoy great health into their nineties!

The truth is, your body is a brilliantly designed machine and if you have any symptoms of ill-health this is a sure sign that your body's chemistry is too acidic. Your symptoms are just a cry for help. This is because the body doesn't just break down one day. Instead, your health erodes slowly over time, finally falling into 'dis-ease'.

When you choose to eat an alkaline diet, you are actually eating foods that are very similar to what man was designed to eat. If you look at what our ancestors ate, you will find a diet rich in fresh fruits, vegetables, legumes, nuts, and fish. Unfortunately, man's diet today is frequently full of foods that are high in unhealthy fats, salt, cholesterol, and acidifying foods.

Although some people think that man's diet changed only recently, the shift from a largely alkaline diet to an acid diet actually began thousands of years ago. Our original diet consisted of foraged fruits, nuts and vegetables, along with whatever meat could be caught. As soon as man started to grow his own food, things started to change. Grains became a popular diet choice, especially after the development of stone tools. Once animals were domesticated, there were dairy products added to the diet, along with an additional amount of meat. Salt began to be added, along with sugar. The end result was a diet that was still much healthier than what many people eat today, but the shift from alkaline to acid had begun.

It's no secret that our modern diet consists of many foods which are not healthy for us. Too much junk food and "fast food" has decreased the quality of our diet. Obesity has become the norm, and along with it a higher incidence of diseases such as diabetes, coronary disease, and cancer. If you want to improve your health and reduce the risk of many diseases, an alkaline diet can help get your body back to basics.

The low carbohydrate and high protein diets doing the rounds these days are an invitation to bad health. All athletes know that if a fit body is to be maintained one should steer completely clear of such diets. Not only do they result in extreme fatigue but also are a disaster where weight management is concerned. Choosing alkaline diets is the only way to live a healthy life as well as shed those extra pounds.

Alkaline diets require one to follow a life style completely opposite of the high protein low carb diets. The high protein diets leave the person following it fatigued and tired. It is for those who lead a stagnant life and want to shed some weight. But the weight that is lost comes back on as soon as one stops the diet. With alkaline diets this is not the case. The diets can be incorporated into ones way of life and within days the results start to show.They require one to eat about 80 % alkalizing foods so as to maintain the alkaline ph of the body to 7.4. High protein diets tend to make the ph of the body acidic as opposed to its natural alkaline tilt. When the body ph becomes acidic it attracts all illnesses and depletes one of energy. An acidic ph also results in rapid degeneration of the human body cells. That leads to a shortened life. One should stay away from these crash diets and look at achieving health and vigor by following alkaline diets instead.

Alkaline diets lead to the body ph maintaining its alkaline nature. The various body functions are carried out smoothly and the immune system of the body stays strong. Under these circumstances one feels energetic as opposed to feeling fatigued. Also the weight shed like this stays off and most importantly the body does not fall sick. In other words they help repel diseases as opposed to high protein diets which seem to attract them. These plans are also very good for those suffering from chronic diseases like arthritis, cancer, migraines, sinusitis and also osteoporosis. Following such a regime while taking medication helps fight these diseases off from the root.

Alkaline diets constitute mostly of fruits and vegetables. One should try and consume green vegetables and sweet fruits so that they make up about 70 to 80 percent of their total food intake. Lemons and melons should also be eaten. Almonds, honey, and olive oil are also high on the list of foods to be consumed for following alkaline diets. Meats and fats should be avoided. All foods that are acidifying like coffee, alcohol, meats, and even certain vegetables like cooked spinach should not form more than 20% of ones diet. Alkaline water is also a must for everyone wanting to improve their diet. At least 6 to 8 glasses of alkaline water can do wonders for your body cleansing. Processed food is all acidic and also high on weight gaining substances and so should be avoided. Beverages like sodas are highly acidic and should not be consumed at all. It takes 32 glasses of water to balance out one glass of soda.

Alkaline diets are for everyone. Each one of us should stop abusing our bodies and look at a healthy and long life by making alkaline diets a part of our life style.

WHAT IS AN ALKALINE DIET?

When foods are eaten and digested, they produce either an acidifying or alkalizing effect within the body. Some people get confused because the actual pH of the food itself doesn't have anything to do with the effect of the food once it is digested. When more alkaline foods are consumed, the body can become slightly alkaline instead of acid. Ideally, the blood pH level should be between 7.35 and 7.45. Foods such as citrus fruits, soy products, raw fruits and vegetables, wild rice, almonds, and natural sweeteners such as Stevia are all good alkaline food choices.

A lot of people have been struggling to find the best diet program fit for them. One of the most common misrepresentation that these people have is their desire to lose weight. They fail to put vital emphasis on how to be healthy. If you want to know the best diet that is perfect for you, then you better make sure it's healthy and is not destroying your body.

THE ALKALINE DIET

Surely, you have encountered an alkaline meal program somewhere online or in some reading materials. What is an alkaline diet and is this diet healthy for you? This diet all started when experts tried considering the pH level of the body. In a person's body, the environment can be acidic or alkaline. Once the pH level is high then the environment is alkaline. In contrary, low pH means the environment is acidic. The body does not have one single pH level rather it can differ depending on the location. The pH level in the stomach is different from the urinary bladder.

This diet is basically all about eating foods which can promote alkaline environment in the body while not eating foods that promote acidity to the body. What could be the reason behind this program? To start off, foods that can promote an alkaline environment in the body, are considered healthy. Examples of these foods include vegetables, fruits, soy products, nuts, legumes, and cereals. If you have noticed, these foods are rich in protein, vitamins, and minerals.

Th other principle of an alkaline diet is to avoid acid foods because these are foods that can make your body at risk for weight gain, heart problems, kidney and liver diseases. Few of the many acid foods include caffeine, foods with high preservatives like canned goods, sodas, fish, meat, alcohol and foods with high sugar content. When you come to think of it, alkaline diet is not unusual for everyone especially when talking about a healthy diet.

REAL DEAL WITH ALKALINE DIET

According to experts, acidic foods can decrease the pH of a person's urine. When the pH is abnormally low kidney stones tend to form. To counteract this situation a person needs to increase the pH through eating alkaline rich foods, that simple.

Since an alkaline diet means avoiding alcohol and any other foods with high acidity, it also means that you will decrease the risk of developing diseases associated with unhealthy diet like diabetes, hypertension, and obesity. Although no exact evidences can prove, some researchers have stated that alkaline diet can reduce the risk of cancer.

In order for alkaline diet to work, you must condition yourself to adhere to the diet program. When it requires you to avoid unhealthy foods and drinks, then you better do it. Water therapy is an excellent alternative drink for soda and alcohol. In addition, so that you will not have a difficult time figuring out which are alkaline and which are acid foods, it is best that you make a list of each category. Perhaps you can research online on what foods are rich in alkaline and those having high acid content. Alkaline foods are not that hard to point because the majority of foods belong to vegetables and fruits classification.

THE ALKALINE DIET - WHAT CAN I EAT ON IT?

The Alkaline Diet is also known as the Alkaline Ash Diet, Alkaline Acid Diet, or the Acid Alkaline Diet.

Doctors such as Robert O. Young, N.D. are championing this diet, and believe a food can be classified as alkaline, acid, or neutral according to pH.

Generally, the diet consists of eating certain citrus, other low sugar fruits, vegetables, tubers, nuts, and legumes.

Grains, dairy products, meat, sugar, alcohol, caffeine, and fungi like mushrooms are to be avoided. By consuming such a diet, it is said that the body maintains a pH of between 7.35 and 7.45 (7.00 is neutral on the pH scale while below 7.00 is acidic).

DIET AND DISEASE

There is some evidence that such a diet is beneficial in preventing osteoporosis and other bone health issues. However, evidence is not strong in supporting the claims that an alkaline diet may prevent or help alleviate conditions such as cancer, fatigue, obesity, or allergies.

There is, however, some evidence that cancer cells grow more quickly in an acidic environment in a laboratory setting. Therefore, a person with a predisposition to or who actually suffers from this disease may want to investigate the effects an alkaline diet have on the body.

Considering the overwhelming rise in many of these types of diseases it is easy to wonder if they are caused by the general condition of a person's internal body environment.

A wider and more scientifically vigorous examination of the Alkaline Diet is in order. However, such scientific scrutiny may be tainted from the beginning by prejudice fomented in a pharmaceutical based health care delivery system.

The theory behind the Alkaline Diet is not widely accepted by the medical community which may be one of the reasons cancer, diabetes, and any number of other terrible diseases are at epidemic levels. The Alkaline Diet, when combined with a physically active, low stress lifestyle certainly deserves more attention from the scientific community if they can keep their bias at bay.

DIET AND DISEASE

It would be relatively simple to see if specific conditions such as blood sugar, blood pressure, cholesterol count, and a person's weight normalize when (and if) their blood pH falls into the desired range. These symptoms occur together so often that the medical community has begun calling it Syndrome X.

If this syndrome is so common, and the protocol for scientific examination so simple, why is the Alkaline Diet still such as mystery as to whether it is beneficial or not?

It may be because there is no money to be made from recommending a specific diet.

Pharmaceutical companies test new drugs because there is a profit to be made if the drug makes it to market. But there is no profit in dietary recommendations therefore such research would fall to the universities and governmental agencies to conduct.

The fact that most of those researchers also work as consultants for the pharmaceutical industry may easily taint their enthusiasm and findings.

GOOD HEALTHY FOOD

SO, WHAT ARE YOU SUPPOSED TO EAT?

It is recommended that you avoid "acidic" foods such as sugar, red meat, shellfish, eggs, dairy, processed and other refined foods, most grains including refined grains, artificial sweeteners, alcohol, caffeine, chocolate, and soda pop.

You should consume raw fruits and vegetables that have a high chlorophyll content such as green leafy vegetables.

The brassica family of vegetables (also known as crucifers) are well represented on the Alkaline Diet and include:

- Broccoli

- Brussels sprouts

- Cabbage

- Cauliflower

- Turnips

- Collard greens

- Kale

- Kohlrabi

- Bok Choi

- Mustard Greens

Other raw vegetables to try on your alkaline diet are:

- Avocado

- Tomato

- Red Beets

- Carrots

- Lima Beans

- Red and black radishes

- Rutabaga

- Egg plant

- Asparagus

- Artichoke

- Lettuce

- Endive

- Cucumber

- Celery

- Peppers

- Zucchini

- Squash

- Spinach

- Peas

- Parsnips

- Onions

HEALTHY FRUIT

The best fruit to consume on the alkaline diet includes:

- Unripe bananas

- Sour cherries

- Fresh coconut

- Figs (either raw or dried)

- Fresh lemon

- Lime

Whether the Alkaline Diet is as good for preventing disease as its proponents claim will have to wait to be seen.

However, following the alkaline diet certainly will keep you within the parameters of what most other medical practitioners and organizations have been claiming to be a healthy diet for many, many years.

ALKALINE DIET FOR HEALTH AND WEIGHT LOSS

There are a lot of crazy diets on the market that promise to help you lose weight. Unfortunately, if you look at the nutritional value of some of these diets, they are often severely lacking. If you need to lose weight, you should do it while eating a diet that is good for your body, so that you will become healthier instead of just thinner. An alkaline diet is a healthy approach to weight loss that will keep you energized, healthy, and motivated to drop the pounds.

UNDERSTANDING THE ALKALINE DIET

An alkaline diet is different from other diets, because it focuses primarily on the effect that foods have on the acidity or the alkalinity of the body. When foods are digested and metabolized by the body, they produce what is commonly referred to as an "alkaline ash" or "acid ash." The original pH of the food doesn't factor into this final effect within the body. In fact, some of the most acidic foods such as citrus fruits actually produce an alkaline effect when eaten. When more alkaline foods are eaten as opposed to acid foods, the pH of the body can be adjusted to an optimum level of approximately 7.3. While this is not extremely alkaline, it is enough to reap many healthful benefits.

USING AN ALKALINE DIET FOR WEIGHT LOSS

Many people attempt fad diets or those which promise quick results in an attempt to lose weight. These diets might produce results in the short term, but over time this can be a very unhealthy way to lose weight. Additionally, many people gain the weight back as soon as they go off their strict diet. When an acid diet is used for weight loss and control, it is more of a lifestyle change. The results may not happen overnight, but it's more likely that the weight will not be gained back. An alkaline diet is rich in foods which are naturally low in calories, such as most vegetables and fruits. Many of the foods that are high in fat and calories are also acidifying, so when these foods are removed from the diet, a natural and healthy weight loss will occur. These foods include red meat, fatty foods, high fat dairy products such as whole milk and cheese, sugar, soda, and alcohol. Once you stop eating these foods, your body will be much healthier, less acid, and you'll also lose weight in the process. Because the diet is healthy, you can stick with it long term. In fact, many people who start an alkaline diet solely for the purpose of losing weight find many other benefits. An increased energy level, resistance to illness, and an overall improvement in health and well-being are among the many benefits you can experience on an alkaline diet.

HOW TO START AN ALKALINE DIET

Many people find that it is easier to start on an alkaline diet by making small changes. Start by slowly reducing the amount of meat, sugar and fat in your diet, while adding fresh fruits, vegetables, healthy fats such as olive oil, almonds, soy products, and natural sweeteners such as Stevia. You'll find over time, your tastes will change and you'll actually start to prefer this kind of diet.

CHOOSING A PROPER ALKALINE DIET MENU

Putting together a successful alkaline diet requires consuming the proper foods and in the proper quantities. Your alkaline diet menu is crucial to the diets success. In this article, you will learn about why alkaline diets are beneficial to our health, how you can successfully implement your diet, and which foods you should place on your alkaline diet menu.

THE HISTORY OF HUMAN DIET

Early man's diet was far different from what we consume today. Early man consumed primarily raw plant based food with occasional, but rare, animal proteins. A typical human diet today consists of much more animal proteins. Also, we now eat a large amount of highly processed and unnatural foods, which are filled with harmful toxins to the body. Excessive salts, fake sugars, and additives increase the acidity of our current diets. This increased intake of acid takes the body out of its natural, healthy, pH balance of 7.3, and does damage to a number of the body's vital processes.

HOW ALKALINE DIETS WORK

By consciously controlling the acid to alkaline balance in your body, you are able to benefit from a wide range of health benefits. Increased energy and weight loss will be immediately noticeable to someone who is recently returning to balance from an overly acidic body. By composing your diet of approximately 75% alkaline foods and only 25% acidic foods, you can return your body to its healthy, natural state. Also, preparing the acidic foods with alkaline water can greatly reduce their acidifying affect on the body. An alkaline diet works to reduce the stress placed on your liver, kidneys, and other organs by having an overly acidic (toxic) body.

YOUR ALKALINE DIET MENU

Below are lists of different foods which are our top recommendations for having an alkaline diet. While foods which are acidic must be ingested for a healthy diet, they are too be lowered back to the levels which our bodies originally adapted to.

Alkaline Fruits:

apples	oranges
bananas	pineapple
blackberries	raisins
dates	

Alkaline Vegetables:

broccoli	eggplant
cabbage	mushrooms
carrots	squash
cauliflower	turnips
celery	

Acidic foods should make up no more than 25% of your diet. Listed below are the types of food which are acidic. Keep in mind that every category listed below has foods which are horribly acidic, but also some which are much more on the alkaline side.

Acidic Foods:

meat

cheese

legumes

grains

nuts

select fruits

select vegetables

A LIST OF ACID, ALKALINE & NEUTRAL FOODS

A balanced diet is one of the keys to good health. One way to ensure a balanced diet is to eat foods from all the food groups; another way is to balance your intake of acidic, or acid-forming, foods with alkaline foods. This helps your body maintain its pH balance, which is essential for proper physiological functioning and preventing disease. Knowing which foods are acid-forming, alkalizing and neutral can help you plan your meals.

ACID-FORMING FOODS

Foods that create an acidic environment in the body include most processed foods, meat and fish, rice, cereal grains, sweeteners and sweetened foods, breads, pastas, cheese, caffeinated drinks, alcohol and condiments. Some nuts and seeds are acid-forming as well. Examples include beef, potato chips, salmon, chicken and pork. Artificial sweeteners, cane and beet sugars, barley syrup, processed honey, maple syrup and molasses are all acidic. Some fruits and vegetables are acid-forming, including most types of beans, dried-sulfured fruits, blueberries and cranberries. Acidic nuts include walnuts, pecans, cashews, pistachios, macadamias, filberts, Brazil nuts and peanuts. Sunflower and pumpkin seeds are also acid-forming. Mustard, ketchup, mayonnaise and vinegar are examples of acidifying condiments. Cola, coffee, sweetened teas, fruit juices beer and wine are acid-forming beverages.

ALKALIZING FOODS

Eating plenty of alkalizing foods helps balance the effects of acidic foods in the body. Most fresh fruits and vegetables are alkalizing. This includes lettuces; all types of potatoes; cruciferous vegetables including broccoli, kale, Brussels sprouts and cauliflower; herbs, such as parsley and dill; and carrots, beets, eggplant and sprouts. Sprouted beans are also alkalizing. Alkalizing fruits include avocados, pears, peaches, cherries, apples, all types of melon, bananas, dates, papayas, figs and grapes. Some dairy products are alkaline, such as buttermilk, raw milk, plain yogurt and acidophilus milk. Amaranth and quinoa are alkalizing grains, and almonds, chestnuts and fresh coconut are alkalizing nuts. Other alkaline foods include honey, kelp, tea and egg yolks.

NEUTRAL FOODS

Neutral foods have neither an acidic nor alkaline effect on the body when consumed. Neutral foods include unsalted, fresh butter; fresh, raw cream; raw cow's milk and whey; and margarine and oils.

CREATING A HEALTHY BALANCE

Just because a food is acid-forming doesn't mean you shouldn't eat it. You need some acid-forming foods in your diet because they are sources of important nutrients such as heart-healthy fatty acids from fish and B vitamins from grains. The key is to eschew unhealthy acid-forming foods like potato chips, refined grains, sweeteners and colas, and choose healthy sources like lean meats, whole grains and plain dairy. Make sure to eat plenty of alkalizing fruits and vegetables. If you follow the U.S. Department of Agriculture's recommendation to fill half your plate with fruits and vegetables at each meal, you're on your way to better health.

THE ALKALINE DIET MYTH

The alkaline diet is also known as the acid-alkaline diet or the alkaline ash diet. It is based around the idea that the foods you eat leave behind an "ash" residue after they have been metabolized. This ash can be acid or alkaline.

Proponents of this diet claim that certain foods can affect the acidity and alkalinity of bodily fluids, including urine and blood. If you eat foods with an acidic ash, they make the body acidic. If you eat foods with an alkaline ash, they make the body alkaline.

Acid ash is thought to make you vulnerable to diseases such as cancer, osteoporosis, and muscle wasting, whereas alkaline ash is considered to be protective. To make sure you stay alkaline, it is recommended that you keep track of your urine using handy pH test strips.

For those who do not fully understand human physiology and are not nutrition experts, diet claims like this sounds rather convincing. However, is it really true? The following will debunk this myth and clear up some confusion regarding the alkaline diet.

But first, it is necessary to understand the meaning of the pH value.

Put simply, the pH value is a measure of how acidic or alkaline something is. The pH value ranges from 0 to 14.

* 0-7 is acidic

* 7 is neutral

* 7-14 is alkaline

For example, the stomach is loaded with highly acidic hydrochloric acid, a pH value between 2 and 3.5. The acidity helps kill germs and break down food.

On the other hand, the human blood is always slightly alkaline, with a pH of between 7.35 to 7.45. Normally, the body has several effective mechanisms (discussed later) to keep the blood pH within this range. Falling out of it is very serious and can be fatal.

EFFECTS OF FOODS ON URINE AND BLOOD PH

Foods leave behind an acid or alkaline ash. Acid ash contains phosphate and sulfur. Alkaline ash contains calcium, magnesium, and potassium.

Certain food groups are considered acidic, neutral, or alkaline.

Acidic: Meats, fish, dairy, eggs, grains, and alcohol.

Neutral: Fats, starches, and sugars.

Alkaline: Fruits, vegetables, nuts, and legumes.

URINE PH

Foods you eat change the pH of your urine. If you have a green smoothie for breakfast, your urine, in a few hours, will be more alkaline than if you had bacon and eggs.

For someone on an alkaline diet, urine pH can be very easily monitored and may even provide instant gratification. Unfortunately, urine pH is neither a good indicator of the overall pH of the body, nor is it a good indicator of general health.

BLOOD PH

Foods you eat do not change your blood pH. When you eat something with an acid ash like protein, the acids produced are quickly neutralized by bicarbonate ions in the blood. This reaction produces carbon dioxide, which is exhaled through the lungs, and salts, which are excreted by the kidneys in your urine.

During the process of excretion, the kidneys produce new bicarbonate ions, which are returned to the blood to replace the bicarbonate that was initially used to neutralize the acid. This creates a sustainable cycle in which the body is able to maintain the pH of the blood within a tight range.

Therefore, as long as your kidneys are functioning normally, your blood pH will not be influenced by the foods you eat, whether they are acidic or alkaline. The claim that eating alkaline foods will make your body or blood pH more alkaline is not true.

ACIDIC DIET AND CANCER

Those who advocate an alkaline diet claim that it can cure cancer because cancer can only grow in an acidic environment. By eating an alkaline diet, cancer cells cannot grow but die.

This hypothesis is very flawed. Cancer is perfectly capable of growing in an alkaline environment. In fact, cancer grows in normal body tissue which has a slightly alkaline pH of 7.4. Many experiments have confirmed this by successfully growing cancer cells in an alkaline environment.

However, cancer cells do grow faster with acidity. Once a tumor starts to develop, it creates its own acidic environment by breaking down glucose and reducing circulation. Therefore, it is not the acidic environment that causes cancer but the cancer that causes the acidic environment.

Even more interesting is a 2005 study by the National Cancer Institute which uses vitamin C (ascorbic acid) to treat cancer. They found that by administering pharmacologic doses intravenously, ascorbic acid successfully killed cancer cells without harming normal cells. This is another example of cancer cells being vulnerable to acidity, as opposed to alkalinity.

In short, there is no scientific link between eating an acidic diet and cancer. Cancer cells can grow in both acidic and alkaline environments.

ACIDIC DIET AND OSTEOPOROSIS

Osteoporosis is a progressive bone disease characterized by a decrease in bone mineral content, leading to lowered bone density and strength and higher risk of a broken bone.

Proponents of the alkaline diet believe that in order to maintain a constant blood pH, the body takes alkaline minerals like calcium from the bones to neutralize the acids from an acidic diet. As discussed above, this is absolutely not true. The kidneys and the respiratory system are responsible for regulating blood pH, not the bones.

In fact, many studies have shown that increasing animal protein intake is positive for bone metabolism as it increases calcium retention and activates IGF-1 (insulin-like growth factor-1) that stimulates bone regeneration. Thus, the hypothesis that an acidic diet causes bone loss is not supported by science.

ACIDIC DIET AND MUSCLE WASTING

Advocates of the alkaline diet believe that in order to eliminate excess acid caused by an acidic diet, the kidneys will steal amino acids (building blocks of protein) from muscle tissues, leading to muscle loss. The proposed mechanism is similar to the one causing osteoporosis.

As discussed, blood pH is regulated by the kidneys and the lungs, not the muscles. Hence, acidic foods like meats, dairy, and eggs do not cause muscle loss. As a matter of fact, they are complete dietary proteins that will support muscle repair and help prevent muscle wasting.

WHAT DID OUR ANCESTORS EAT?

A number of studies have examined whether our pre-agricultural ancestors ate net acidic or net alkaline diets. Very interestingly, they found that about half of the hunter-gatherers ate net acid-forming diets, while the other half ate net alkaline-forming diets.

Acid-forming diets were more common as people moved further north of the equator. The less hospitable the environment, the more animal proteins they ate. In more tropical environments where fruits and vegetables were abundant, their diet became more alkaline.

From an evolutionary perspective, the theory that acidic or protein-rich diets cause diseases like cancer, osteoporosis, and muscle loss is not valid. Half of the hunter-gatherers were eating net acid-forming diets, yet, they had no evidence of such degenerative diseases.

It is worth noting that there is no one-size-fits-all diet that works for everyone, which is why Metabolic Typing is so helpful in determining your optimal diet. Due to our genetic variances, some people will benefit from an acidic diet, some an alkaline diet, and some in between. Thus the saying: one man's food can be another man's poison.

It is true that many people who have switched to an alkaline diet see significant health improvements. However, do bear in mind that other reasons may be at work:

    * Most of us do not eat enough vegetables and fruits. According to the

Center for Disease and Prevention, only 9% of Americans eat enough vegetables and 13% enough fruits. If you switch to an alkaline diet, you are automatically eating more vegetables and fruits. After all, they are very rich in phytochemicals, antioxidants, and fiber which are essential to good health. When you eat more vegetables and fruits, you are probably eating less processed foods too.

* Eating less dairy and eggs will benefit those who are lactose-intolerant or have a food sensitivity to eggs, which is rather common among the general population.

* Eating less grains will benefit those who are gluten-sensitive or have leaky gut or an autoimmune disease.

ALKALINE WATER

One last point worth mentioning is that many people believe that drinking alkaline water (pH of 9.5 vs. pure water's pH of 7.0.) is healthier based on similar reasoning as the alkaline diet. Anyhow, it is not true. Water that is too alkaline can be detrimental to your health and lead to nutritional disequilibrium.

If you drink alkaline water all the time, it will neutralize your stomach acid and raise the alkalinity of your stomach. Over time, it will impair your ability to digest food and absorb nutrients and minerals. With less acidity in the stomach, it will also open the door for bacteria and parasites to get into your small intestine.

The bottom line is that alkaline water is not the answer to good health. Do not be fooled by marketing gimmicks. Instead, invest in a good water filtration system for your home. Clean, filtered water is still the best water for your body.

BENEFITS OF ALKALINE DIET FOR DIABETICS

HUMAN BODY DESIGN AND ALKALINE DIET

The human body is, to some degree, alkaline by design. By maintaining it alkaline we allow it to run at an ideal level. Nevertheless, millions of reactions of our metabolism yield acidic wastes as end products. When we consume an excessive amount of acid-producing foods and not enough alkaline-forming foods we aggravate the body acid intoxication. If we let these acid-wastes build-up throughout the body, a disorder known as acidosis develops over time.

Acidosis will progressively debilitate our body vital functions, if we do not quickly take corrective actions. Acidosis, or body over-acidity, is in fact one of the leading causes of human aging. It makes our body highly vulnerable to the series of the deadly degenerative chronic diseases, such as diabetes, cancer, arthritis, as well as heart diseases.

For this reason, the biggest challenge we humans have to face to protect our lives is actually to find the right way to reduce the production, and to maximize the elimination of the body acidic wastes. To avoid acidosis and the age-related diseases, and to continue running at its highest level possible, our body needs a healthy lifestyle. This lifestyle should include regular exercises, a balanced nutrition, a clean physical environment, and a way of living that brings the lowest stress possible. A healthy lifestyle allows our body to keep its acid waste content at the lowest level possible.

The alkaline diet, also known as the pH miracle diet, seems to fit the best the design of the human body. This is mainly because it helps neutralize the acid wastes and allows flushing them out from the body. People should look at alkaline diet as general dietary boundaries for humans to abide by. The persons who have particular health issues and special medical diets might better accommodate those diets to alkaline diet boundaries.

ALKALINE DIET BENEFITS FOR DIABETICS

The miracle alkaline diet will help improve the overall health of the persons suffering from diabetes. As it does for other human beings, alkaline diet will help boost their body physiology and metabolism, as well as their immune system. This diet will allow diabetics to have a better control on their blood sugar. It is also going to help not only in reducing their weight gain and the risks of cardiovascular diseases, but also in keeping their cholesterol level low.

In fact, the alkaline diet allows a better management of diabetes and, as a result, it helps diabetics avoid more easily the degenerative diseases connected to their condition. So by following an alkaline diet, despite their health situation, diabetics can, at the same time, live healthier and extend considerably their life expectancy.

DIABETICS ACID-ALKALINE FOOD CHART

In general, people who want to follow an alkaline diet need to select their daily food items from an 'Acid-Alkaline Foods Chart'. We recently published a 'Diabetics Acid-Alkaline Food Chart'. The use of this specific chart allows diabetics to conform to both the alkaline diet rule and the glycemic index rule.

The alkaline diet rule sets general nutritional guidelines. According to this diet plan, our daily food intake should be composed of a minimum of 80 percent of alkaline-forming foods, and of no more than 20 percent of acidifying food products. Additionally, the diet highlights that the more alkaline a food item is, the better it is actually; and on the other hand the more acidifying a food product is, the worse it should be for the human body.

As for the glycemic index rule, it divides foods into four main categories with respect to their ability to raise the blood sugar. This ability is now measured by the glycemic index GI that ranges from 0 to 100.

(1) Foods that contain almost no carbohydrates and that have, in consequence, a negligible glycemic index (GI~0); diabetics may take them freely.

(2) Foods containing carbohydrates with a low glycemic index (GI 55 or less); people with diabetes should eat these products with some precaution.

(3) Foods that have carbohydrates of high glycemic index (GI 56 or more); diabetics must, so far as possible, exclude them from their diet.

(4) Processed foods; diabetics will need to consult the manufacturers' labels to figure out their particular glycemic index values.

TOP 10 HEALTHIEST ALKALINE DIET FOODS

Ever heard of alkaline diet foods? If not, it is high time you do. Work pressure, home making, maintaining personal and professional relations is taking a toll on everyone's food habits, resulting in more than 70% of the present generation suffering from acidity and heartburn. Every third person seems to be complaining of gastric problems, indigestion and acid reflux. All of this is due to the imbalance in the acid-alkaline pH of foods that consumed these days, where you simply grab something and rush to work. Fast foods, sodas and the like are being consumed left, right and center by the young generation, thus giving rise to deficiency in minerals, vitamins and nutrition.

Alkaline diets have been found to be extremely beneficial for optimum health. You can keep chronic ailments such as acidity, osteoporosis, and generalized weakness at arm's length with foods rich in alkaline content. Alkaline foods are important since the pH of human blood is slightly more alkaline. This makes it necessary that we have more of alkaline pH than acidic content in the body.

WHAT ARE THE BENEFITS OF ALKALINE DIETS?

Alkaline diet foods have a plethora of benefits such as:

* Improved resistance   * Strong teeth and Bones

* Vibrant temperament   * Easy Digestion

* Increased Alertness

Alkaline diet foods are vital to maintain the pH levels of blood at an optimum of 7. Alkaline foods are mostly vegetarian foods consisting of fresh foods and vegetables.

LISTED HERE ARE THE TOP 10 HEALTHIEST ALKALINE FOODS FOR NUTRITIONAL BENEFITS:

1. Spinach and Greens - Spinach has been found to contain maximum benefits and is highly alkaline. It can be consumed raw or cooked with equal effect. Other leafy green vegetables such as lettuce, fenugreek leaves, basil etc. also are extremely good as alkaline foods. They also contain a lot of minerals and vitamins as an added advantage.

2. Cucumber - Raw cucumber is not only a zero-calorie vegetable, it is highly alkaline when consumed raw. It is delicious and contains a host of nutritional benefits. Cucumber improves overall digestion and keeps your skin fresh and glowing. It contains healthy alkaline water that helps in flushing out unwanted wastes from the body.

3. Banana - Banana can be considered a whole food due its numerous dietary advantages. It gives instant energy and is hugely alkaline. In fact, if you are suffering from severe acidic problems, a banana diet can work wonders in reducing the burning sensation and indigestion remarkably. Bananas have healthy sugar content and can be consumed by anyone irrespective of his health condition.

4. Celery - Celery is a delicious alkaline food that can help you immensely in keeping your pH levels at normal range of 7. When half-cooked, it gives maximum nutritional value and can be eaten as fresh salad too.

5. Broccoli - Broccoli is one of the most nutritious and alkaline foods that has proved itself time and again. It is easily digestible and is a rich source of valuable minerals such as carotene and calcium. These minerals help in improving immunity and combat diseases in a remarkable manner.

6. Avocado - This wonder fruit is a rich source of alkaline food and has an overall benefit in maintaining good health. Avocado improves your hemoglobin content and is extremely beneficial in restoring normalcy in a disease affected body.

7. Capsicum - Capsicum, also known as bell pepper is a rich anti oxidant and can be useful whether eaten cooked or raw. It is not only of high alkaline and nutritional value, it is also very delicious and adds taste to any dishes that are prepared with capsicum for flavor.

8. Potato Skin - Although potato is found to be acidic in nature, potato skin is very rich in alkaline content. Raw potato juice is found to be very useful in reducing the acidic content in the stomach.

9. Soy beans - Soy beans and soy milk are greatly alkaline and can be used as nutritional alkaline foods.

10. Cold Milk - Cold milk is found to have high alkaline content and is often recommended to combat heartburn and acid reflux disorders.

Alkaline diet foods are becoming very popular among health conscious individuals who have realized their great benefits and high nutritional value.

ALKALINE PROMOTING FOODS

Our blood pH should be maintained at a slightly alkaline level in order to keep us healthy. We help our bodies to maintain this pH balance by eating more alkaline-forming foods and fewer acid-forming foods.

Unfortunately, due to decades of societal changes, millions of dollars of marketing, and even technological advances, humans are facing more dietary based health challenges than ever before. It's really no coincidence that the rapidly growing numbers of obesity, diabetes, cancer, and cardiovascular disease happen to correlate almost exactly with the rise in consumption of acid-forming foods like sugars, trans fats, fast food, refined food and white breads. At the same time, we've dramatically decreased the consumption of fresh, whole foods like vegetables.

All of that, combined with a long list of other environmental factors like stress, lack of sleep and pharmaceutical drugs, make it not all that surprising that more and more people are being diagnosed with chronic, degenerative illness or other potentially fatal conditions for which modern medicine claims to have no known cure.

When we consume acid-forming foods, the body brings our blood pH back into balance by releasing alkaline-rich minerals like calcium, phosphorus and magnesium into the bloodstream. If we are getting enough alkaline-forming foods in our daily diet, then the body has easy access to these minerals, but if we aren't consuming enough alkaline-forming foods, then the body is forced to pull these essential minerals from our bones, teeth and organs. That can weaken the immune system, resulting in fatigue and a greater vulnerability to viruses and disease.

As our pH level is partially determined by the mineral density of the foods one eats, it's important to consume plenty of alkaline foods. Ideally, a balanced diet should include about 60 to 80 percent alkaline-forming foods, and 20 to 40 percent acid-forming foods. Maintaining an acid alkaline balance is essential for our good health, not only for optimal pH levels, but for many other reasons as well.

Of course, in order to follow a diet that includes 60 to 80 percent alkaline foods, you need to know exactly what those foods are.

1. BEETS

Beets and other vegetables tend to be richer in minerals, and they're also one of the best foods for helping to raise pH levels. Plus, it offers a wealth of other health benefits too, as one of the few sources of a phytonutrient known as betalain, which is believed to offer cancer prevention properties.

If you don't like that earthy taste, peel off the skins and add them in a smoothie. Otherwise, they're great fresh steamed or as a salad topper too.

2. SEA VEGETABLES

Sea vegetables like kelp, dulse, nori, and wakame are excellent alkaline foods as some of the most mineral-rich foods on Earth, packed with potassium and magnesium as well as vitamin A, C and K. You can use sea veggies by adding them to a soup or salad, and, if you're avoiding gluten or grains, you can use Nori wraps as a substitute for a grain-based wrap.

3. HEMP SEEDS

Hemp has often been classified as one of nature's most perfect foods, and it's probably no surprise that it's considered to be an alkaline food as well. That's because it's loaded with chlorophyll, which is known to be alkalizing, helping to combat acidity while normalizing the body's pH, as well as aiding in cleansing, healing, and detoxification. These tiny seeds are also powerhouses of dietary fiber, antioxidants, vitamins and minerals, like calcium, vitamin D, vitamin B, vitamin E, iron, magnesium, zinc, copper, manganese, and phosphorus.

Add hemp seeds to a smoothie, yogurt, oatmeal, salad, or simply snack on them alone. To enjoy the benefits, just be sure that they are 100% raw and organic like these ones you can buy from Amazon.

4. SPIRULINA

Spirulina is a form of sea algae, but it's not a sea vegetable. This superfood is hard to beat when it comes to alkalizing the blood, and on top of that, it contains 80 percent of the daily recommended value for iron, most of your requirements for B vitamins, and, it's loaded with vitamin A – containing more than 800 percent of your daily needs. Spirulina is also one of the few foods with a natural GLA content. Gamma Linolenic Acid. GLA is difficult to find in a food source, and typically has to be created by the body. It offers anti-inflammatory properties and has been found to help combat chronic inflammation, eczema, dermatitis, asthma, rheumatoid arthritis, atherosclerosis, diabetes, obesity and even cancer.

5. GARLIC

One of the most powerful superfoods of all, garlic is often at the top of foods lists for improving overall health, and it's also a top alkaline-forming food. Being highly alkaline, it helps regulate pH, but it also offers a host of other benefits, including lowering blood pressure and cholesterol, helping to prevent the flu or a cold, reducing the risk of heart disease, preventing cancer and fighting off fungal and bacterial infections.

Garlic can add flavor and medicinal benefits to all sorts of dishes, like pasta sauce, salsas, homemade salad dressings and more. To maximize its benefits, before consuming or adding to a dish, chop it up and let it to rest for about 10 minutes. This allows its beneficial, health-promoting allicin content to form.

6. CAYENNE PEPPER

As part of a family of potent peppers that contain enzymes essential to endocrine function, cayenne is considered to be one of the most alkalizing foods. It's known for its antibacterial properties as well as being an excellent source of vitamin A, helping to fight off harmful free radicals that lead to stress and disease. An added bonus? Eating cayenne peppers is also believed to help speed up the metabolism, promoting weight loss.

7. LEMONS

While you might think that lemons are acidic, they're actually one of the most alkaline forming foods there is. This sour fruit provides powerful and immediate relief for hyperacidity and virus-related conditions, as well as coughs, colds, flu and heartburn too. Adding a squeeze of lemon to your water is a great way to add flavor to help ensure you're getting at least eight glasses of day, and drinking a glass of lemon water first thing in the morning is a great way to begin your day by getting those pH levels balanced out.

8. CELERY

Celery is an outstanding alkalizing food. It's filled with vitamin C, vitamin K, natural electrolytes and lots of water, all important for helping to restore the body's balance, and preventing the loss of electrolytes which can lead to excess inflammation. It also contains a lesser-known nutrient, phthalides, which have been shown to lower cholesterol, as well as coumarin, known to inhibit a number of different cancers. Munching on celery is also known to help reduce high blood pressure, further reducing the risk of heart disease.

Eat celery on its own, or chop it up and add it to a stew. It also makes a great base for juices and soups.

9. SPROUTED ALMONDS

Almonds, in general, are an alkalizing food, but sprouted almonds are even better. That's because the soaking and sprouting process helps to reduce some of the nut's acidic properties. When nuts are soaked and germinated, their pH increases, which makes them more alkaline as well as making them easier to digest and helping the body to assimilate the vitamin E, potassium, and magnesium.

Sprouted almonds can be used just like you'd use ordinary almonds. They make a great protein-packed snack on their own, or you can even use them to replace meat by grinding them into a healthy burger.

10. BROCCOLI

Broccoli is one of those vegetables that offers so much nutritional value and so many benefits that it is a must to include in your diet for better health. It's been proven time and again to be amazingly powerful for supporting the digestive and cardiovascular systems, inhibiting cancers, supporting the skin, immune system and metabolism. Eating it steamed or raw makes it an even more alkaline, nutritious food.

In addition to using broccoli in a stir-fry, you can steam it with other vegetables, use it in juices or smoothies, add it to a salad or eat it raw on its own.

11. AVOCADO

Avocado is a powerful, alkaline, nutrient-dense superfood. It contains healthy fats that can help prevent hunger pangs in between meals by keeping you feeling fuller and satisfied longer, and, thanks to its high content of oleic acid, it can help to lower total cholesterol, while raising levels of "good" or HDL cholesterol, and reducing "bad," or LDL cholesterol. Oleic acid also works to slow the development of heart disease and even speed up the metabolism to support weight loss. It also offers a host of other nutrients that offer anti-cancer, anti-inflammatory and blood sugar benefits.

12. BELL PEPPERS

Bell peppers offer antioxidant superpower, are sweet, crunchy and can be used in almost any meal raw, roasted or grilled. This highly alkaline food contains flavonoids, carotenoids and hydroxycinnamic acids. In fact, bell peppers contain more than 30 different members of the carotenoid nutrient family – the only other food that comes close is the tomato. Bell peppers have been linked to a lower risk of cancer, inflammation, diabetes, cardiovascular disease and more.

There are lots of ways to sneak more bell peppers into your diet. They are ideal to toss into a stir-fry, for topping a pizza, transforming into stuffed bell peppers and chopping up into scrambled eggs.

13. CUCUMBER

This alkalizing food is 95% water. That makes it an astonishingly hydrating food, and cucumbers are also loaded with an incredible amount of antioxidants, including lignans, which have a significantly strong, scientifically proven reduced risk of cardiovascular disease and cancer, including ovarian, uterine, breast and prostate cancers.

Cucumbers make the perfect base for an alkaline soup, juice or smoothie too, delivering, in addition to the above, a host of vitamins and minerals like vitamin C and K, as well as calcium, potassium, phosphorus, iron, magnesium, copper, selenium and zinc.

14. BOK CHOY

Bok choy is a good source of vitamin A, C, and K as well as fiber and folate. It also contains phenolic compounds known to help battle against free radical damage and fight cancer cells, along with healthy omega-3 fatty acids.

You can add bok choy to stews, stir-frys and soups, or shred it and use it raw in wraps or salads.

15. CANTALOUPE

This highly alkaline-forming, low-oxalate, nutrient-dense fruit contains 90 percent of the recommended daily allowance of vitamin C and 129 percent of the recommended daily allowance of vitamin B6. It's also an outstanding source of carotenes and potassium.

16. KALE

Kale may be a trendy superfood these days, but with good reason. It's considered to be one of the most alkaline foods and is also widely known for its ability to aid the body in detoxification, lower total cholesterol and fight cancer. Similar to spinach, it has an astoundingly high amount of vitamin K, as well as vitamins C and A, in addition to its chlorophyll content, which as mentioned, is well-known to be alkalizing, helping to combat acidity while normalizing the body's pH, as well as aiding in cleansing, healing and detoxification.

You can use raw kale in a salad, add it to a soup (It doesn't fall apart into moist strings like spinach), toss it into a smoothie, boil it, and turn it into kale chips for a super healthy snack.

17. SPINACH

All leafy greens are important to include on an alkaline diet, and spinach is a favorite as it's so simple to use, extremely versatile and a nutritional powerhouse that's one of the top alkaline foods. As with all green veggies, it's rich in chlorophyll too. Spinach is also packed with vitamins K and A, folate, iron, manganese, magnesium, fiber and more.

It's incredibly easy to add more spinach to your diet – use it in smoothies and juices, add it to scrambled eggs, make a spinach salad, use it as a pizza topping, in sandwiches, tacos, and so on and so on.

18. COCONUT OIL

Coconut oil is the only alkaline forming oil. It contains healthy fats known to benefit the body, rather than harm it. Experts recommend using raw, virgin coconut oil as a replacement for vegetable oils that are chemically processed.

19. MATCHA GREEN TEA

Matcha green tea contains 40 times the antioxidants that regular green tea has, and it's loaded with chlorophyll. Not only is it super alkalizing, but it can help to reduce inflammation, balance blood sugar cravings and improve your mood.

20. WATERMELON

Watermelon has a pH level of 9.0, which means it's very alkaline. It's also 92% water, so it's super hydrating and thirst quenching, and it is an excellent source of vitamin C, lycopene, and beta-carotene.

Enjoy a slice on a hot summer's day, add frozen watermelon cubes to a smoothie, toss it into a salad, or even grill it on skewers.

21. RAISINS

Raisins and other dried fruit, like apricots, a high on the alkaline scale. They're also an excellent source of fiber, vitamins B1 and B6 and antioxidants. Plus, they make a convenient, nutritious snack.

22. RADISHES

Radishes come in a wide variety of colors, shapes, and sizes. But no matter what type of radish you choose, all are highly alkaline-forming. Radishes are a rich source of vitamin C and a good source of calcium too. As they're very low in calories, munching on them can be a great way to keep your mouth busy when you're trying to lose weight.

23. FRESH HERBS

All fresh herbs are considered alkalizing. Parsley, in particular, is very rich in alkaline compounds, as is basil and dried dill weed. No matter what you choose, simply using more fresh, dried herbs in your meals is a great way to follow a more alkaline diet.

24. HERBAL TEA

Just about every herb, as well as water, is alkalizing, which means herbal teas are alkalizing too. Note that herbal teas DON'T contain caffeine, which is an acid-forming substance. Some of the best alkalizing herbal teas are dandelion root tea, chamomile, ginger, and peppermint.

25. ALKALINE WATER

Drinking enough water is essential for good health, as dehydration leads to fatigue and a host of other problems. Alkaline water can help even more than drinking regular water, as it helps deliver nutrients more efficiently, which means you'll enjoy more energy all day long.

Every living cell in your body is made from the food that you eat so eat like your life depends on it because it does!

7-DAY ALKALINE DIET MEAL PLAN

If you consistently eat junk food then you will have junk cells and a junk body. This does not mean that you will be fat or overweight but it means you will have poor quality cells and you will be at higher risk of illness and disease. Eat good quality organic, real whole foods from the earth and lean cuts of meat & organic dairy with no antibiotics or hormones to give your cells the best quality nutrients to build a strong healthy body.

Here is a meal plan with a lot of variety so you have options. This meal plan does include meat, dairy and eggs so if you are a vegetarian then you will have to make substitutions to satisfy your needs.

If you have a favorite meal or snack you can have that for 3-4 days you do not have to change your meals every day. You also have to adjust for your own personal likes, dislikes and food allergies. I recommend using all organic foods, farm raised, grass fed and local farmers with no antibiotics, hormones, pesticides or chemicals. To have healthy cells and a healthy body you must eat quality food.

MEAL PLAN BASED ON 1500-2000 CALORIES A DAY.

Adjust portion sizes so your calorie total fits within your personal daily caloric intake.

DAY 1

Breakfast: Scrambled Egg Whites, Sautéed Collard Greens, Turkey Bacon, Brown Rice, Green tea/w Lemon

Snack: Half-cup of organic low-fat cottage cheese with a half-cup of fresh berries

Lunch: Grilled Chicken Breast/ Garlic Spinach/ Half cup baked yam

Snack: Orange

Snack: Celery and Carrot Sticks with Hummus

Dinner: Albacore Tuna Chopped Salad

Dessert: Honey Dew Melon

Water: Half your body weight in ounces 87ounces = -2.5 liters of Water

DAY 2

Breakfast: Oatmeal Egg White Breakfast Frittata/ topped w Cottage Cheese, Berries and Apple Sauce and side salad with Lemon & Olive Oil or Low fat Balsamic Dressing

Green tea/w Lemon

Snack: Grapefruit

Lunch: Turkey Chili/3 or 4 multi grain or whole wheat crackers

Snack: Mixed Grilled Vegetables with Olive Oil

Snack: All Fresh Green Juice/Smoothie (2-3 handfuls of spinach, 1 Apple, 1 Lemon, thumb-size of Ginger, ice & water)

Dinner: Asian Chicken or Vegetable Stir-fry

Dessert: Cantaloupe

Water: Half of your bodyweight in ounces – 2.5

DAY 3

Breakfast: Veggie Egg White Omelet (Spinach, Mushrooms, Red & Yellow Peppers) Turkey

Sausage Patties/ one slice of Ezekiel bread with all-fruit blueberry jam

Green tea/w Lemon

Snack: Half-cup organic Greek Yogurt with Berries

Lunch: Turkey Ezekiel Sandwich Wrap (mustard, Lettuce, Sprouts, Cucumber, Tomato, Hummus)

Snack: Kale Salad (Dried Cranberries & Walnuts, Olive Oil & Lemon)

Snack: Organic Popcorn (Air Popped) or Apple / Banana

Dinner: Baked Romano Wild Trout/ Spaghetti squash/ Broccoli Parmesan

Dessert: Mixed Berries

Water: Half of your bodyweight in ounces- 2.5 to 3 Liters of water

DAY 4

Breakfast: Whole Wheat Breakfast Burrito with Egg whites, Ground Turkey, Tomatoes, Onions & Side Salad

Green tea/w Lemon

Snack: Orange, Apple or Banana (Piece of Fruit)

Lunch: Grilled Chicken/Broccoli Parmesan/ Baked Butternut Squash

Snack: Pita Chips and Hummus

Snack: Super Rich Green Smoothie (3 Handfuls of Spinach, 1 Apple, 1 Lemon with ¼ Lemon peel, 1 handful of Blueberries, 5 Strawberries, 1 Kiwi, 1 cup of Water, 5 ice cubes) in blender or vitamix machine

Dinner: Grilled Halibut with Mango Salsa/ Roasted Asparagus

Dessert: Bowl of Mixed Berries

Water: 2.5 Liters of water

DAY 5

Breakfast: Millet Porridge with cinnamon flax seeds & mixed berries

(Alkaline breakfast cereal, oatmeal, spelt and other grains are acidic)

Green tea/w Lemon

Snack: Orange Supreme Smootihe (2 cups of carrots, 1 Orange, 1 lemon or lime, 1 thumbsize of Ginger, 1 cup of water, 5 ice cubes)

Lunch: Turkey Meatloaf*/ Sautéed Collard Greens/ Sweet Potato

Snack: Cucumber & Tomato Salad with Feta Cheese, Olive Oil & Lemon

Snack: Smoked salmon/Lemon/ Multigrain crackers Dinner: Curried Chicken Salad*

Dinner: Chinese Chicken Salad*

Dessert: Grapes & Walnuts

Water: 2.5 Liters of water

DAY 6

Breakfast: Smoked Salmon or Fresh Wild Salmon /Poached Eggs/ Sautéed Spinach or Side Salad

Green tea/w Lemon

Snack: Piece of Fruit (Honeydew/Cantaloupe/Apple/Orange/Grapefruit/Mango/Mixed Berries)

Lunch: Canned Tuna Sandwich with Tomatoes, onions, Olive Oil & Lemon on Whole Wheat Pita with Lettuce & Tomatoes

Snack: Cucumber/ Carrots/ Celery stalks/ Hummus

Snack: Steamed Broccoli & Red Peppers with Lemon & Olive Oil

Dinner: Baked Lemon Herb Chicken/ Pear Pine Nut Salad

Dessert: Mixed Fruit Salad

Water: Half of your bodyweight in ounces 2.5 Liters

DAY 7

Breakfast: Blueberry and Banana Buckwheat Pancakes with Organic Turkey Bacon or Turkey Sausage

Green tea/w Lemon

Snack: Two hard boiled eggs, mashed and seasoned with a dash of salt and pepper

Lunch: Turkey Burger

Snack: Roasted Brussel Sprouts with Onions, Olive Oil & Lemon

Snack: Grapefruit

Dinner: Broiled Lemon Garlic Sea Bass/ Roasted Acorn Squash/ Lemon Green Beans

Dessert: Watermelon or Bowl of Mixed Berries

Water: Half of your bodyweight in ounces 2.5 Liters

MEAL PLAN MACRONUTRIENT AND CALORIC BREAKDOWN

This does not have to be exact, it is just a breakdown to give you a guideline of the amount of calories and macronutrients (Healthy Fat, Carbohydrates & Protein) you should be having per meal.

Breakfast: 30grams Protein, 12grams Fat, 40-60 grams Carbohydrates

400-500 Calories

Snack: 14 grams Protein, 6 grams Fat, 20 grams of Carbohydrates

100-200 Calories

Lunch: 30 grams Protein, 12grams Fat, 40-60 grams Carbohydrates

400 -500 Calories

Snack: 14grams Protein, 6 grams Fat, 20 grams of Carbohydrates

100-200 Calories

Snack: 14grams Protein, 6 grams Fat, 20 grams of Carbohydrates

100-200 Calories

Dinner: 30 grams of protein, 12 grams Fat, 25 -50 grams Carbohydrates

300-400 Calories

OPTIMAL HEALTH SUPPLEMENT RECOMMENDATIONS

1) **Multivitamin**– I recommend an all natural wholefood multivitamin. Your vitamins should come from Whole Foods. If the label does not say that it is coming from whole foods then it may be synthetic which is chemically made in a lab and the nutrients do not come from food. Your Vitamins should be ISO9000 certified and NSF Certified. Your Multivitamin should be free of any additives.

All vitamins come from fresh whole, raw foods so the closest to the original form is the best quality for your body. I recommend to juice green vegetables or take a green supplement like Macrogreens.

Macrogreens & other green supplements often have the nutritional value of 3-5 servings of fruits and vegetables. They are simply dehydrated fruits & vegetables but read the labels to make sure there are no additional ingredients.

1) **Probiotics**– are healthy bacteria that help protect the stomach, help you with digestion of food and help you strengthen your immune system. Probiotics are live healthy bacteria that naturally occur in milk and other foods but are destroyed through pasteurization. The healthy bacteria in your stomach gets destroyed when you take antibiotics and you must replace it to strengthen your immune system. (I recommend Bio-K or Udo's Probiotics or Kombucha but there are also other great sources)

2) **Enzymes** – enzymes come from plants and are used to help you digest your food and absorb nutrients. (I recommend Udo's Enzymes or Wholesome Fast Food)

3) **Omega-3 Fatty Acid** – Essential Fat 80% of American's are deficient. Necessary for proper brain function, building block to many hormones, oxygen transport system to the muscle cell. (Carlson's Brand Fish Oil or Udo's Oil 3.6.9 Blend)

5 NUTRITION TIPS

1) **Prepare Your Meals at Home**: Prepare your meals at home and bring them with you. You will be less stressed out and you will save time and money if you plan your meals in advance and bring them with you.

2) **3 Servings of Green Vegetables a Day**: Have 3 servings of green vegetables a day. Greens help alkalinize the body which means they help strengthen your immune system & decrease your risk of illness and disease. They are also loaded with fiber to help you with digestion and elimination. Greens are also loaded with minerals, vitamins, nutrients and phytonutrients to help all of your cells function at their best. Green Smoothies and Green Juices can help you increase your green vegetable intake.

3) **Water**: Half your body weight and drink that number in ounces of water a day. If you weight 150lbs you should be drinking 75oz which is about 4-5 small 16oz bottles. Your body weight is 60% water and every living cell in your body requires water to function. Chronic dehydration can lead to acid reflux, heart burn, constipation, poor digestion, headaches, migraines, arthritis, joint pain and much more.

4) **Green Tea**: Have 2-3 Cups of Green Tea a day. There are antioxidants in Green tea called Catechins that slow down and stop the growth of cancer cells. Many research studies have shown that 2-3 cups of green tea a day can decrease your risk of all cancers. Green Tea also helps alkalinize the body and strengthen the immune system.

5) **Listen To Your Body**: We are all biogenetically unique which means one meal plan does not serve all. One man's food can be another man's poison. If you eat a particular type of food and you feel

fatigued, bloated, break out in a rash or have indigestion then listen to your body and adjust your meals. Healthy eating is also a journey to find what foods work best with your body chemistry so you can function at your best.

Healthy Living is a choice you make every day and it's a way of life!

THE ACIDITY OF FOOD

There was a widely held belief that eating certain foods that were acidic would lead to stomach ulcers. Indeed for many years doctors would advise patients that were diagnosed with ulcers to avoid certain foods. People who suffer from heartburn also often try to find something in their diet that is adding acid to their stomach. But a closer look at the acidity of foods and the events that go on in the stomach during a meal shows that foods are not the source of many upset stomachs. Acidity is measured on a scale from 1 to 14 and is expressed as a pH value. A pH of 1 is very acidic, a pH of 14 is very weakly acidic or more commonly referred to as being very basic. A food or drink that has a pH of 7 is neutral, neither acidic nor basic. Distilled water has a pH of 7. Foods or drinks that have a pH below 7 are acidic, and those above pH 7 are basic. On the acidic side of the scale, a lower number means more acidic. A pH of 2 is more acidic than a pH of 3. On the basic side, a higher number means more basic. A pH of 10 is more basic than a pH of 9.

The 1-14 pH scale is not a linear scale however, which makes it a bit more complicated to understand. The pH scale is in fact a logarithmic scale. So a food that has a pH of 2 is 1 unit of pH different than a food with a pH of 3, but in fact is 10 times more acidic. If two foods have pH's that are 2 pH units apart, their acidity is 100 times different.

Just about all foods that we eat are acidic - have a pH between 2 and 7. But the stomach is also a very acid place. Once we start eating, acid is secreted into the stomach to start the digestion process. The secretions mix with the food in the stomach and the resulting mixture can have a pH of 1.0-3.0 - very acidic. So when you eat carrots that have a pH of 6, they end up in the stomach that can be 10,000 times more acidic. Even acidic foods such as oranges, lemons or wines are not as acidic as the as normal stomach contents.

It is often not the food we eat that causes acidity problems in the stomach, but an over production of acid that is secreted into the stomach following a meal. Some foods can in fact help reduce the acidity in the stomach by neutralizing (reducing) some of the acidity. Foods higher on the pH scale will tend to do this. The beneficial effects of milk probably has more to do with reducing the acidity in the stomach contents than its reported coating of stomach lining effects.

TABLE 1: PH OF SOME COMMON FOODS

eggs 7.6 - 8.0 — Bananas 4.5 - 4.7

Corn 6.0 - 6.5 — Carrots 4.9 - 5.3

Oysters 6.1 - 6.6 — Cherries 3.2 - 4.0

Cow's milk 6.3 - 6.6 — Oranges 3.0 - 4.0

Wheat flour 5.5 - 6.5 — Soft drinks 2.0 - 4.0

Potatoes 5.6 - 6.0 — Wines 2.8 - 3.8

Squash 5.0 - 5.4 — Lemons 2.2 - 2.4

DIABETES, SUGAR AND HEART DISEASE

Heart disease is one of the most common complications of diabetes. Indeed, most diabetics who fail to control their blood glucose levels are killed by heart disease.

In addition, if you are diabetic then there is an 85 percent chance that you also suffer from high cholesterol and blood pressure levels, and this increases the risk of heart disease. If you smoke, you up the risk even further.

In order to beat diabetes and avoid heart disease you need-besides giving up smoking, reducing your cholesterol and getting your blood pressure under control-to reduce the amount of glucose your digestive system produces by limiting the amount of sugar you ingest.

But how much sugar should you ingest on a daily basis? What are the limits?

CALORIES FROM ADDED SUGAR

The number of calories each of us requires on a daily basis depends on our age, height, gender and level of activity. On average, however, a healthy adult needs 2,000 calories a day and a child 1,200 calories.

Natural foodstuffs, such as fruits and vegetables, contain sugar. But it seems that this is not enough for most of us. Sugar is added by diners, chefs and food processors. How much of this added sugar do we need?

Not much. In fact, this added sugar is a major problem with our modern Western diet.

In March 2014, the Journal of the American Medical Association published findings from the National Health and Nutrition Examination Survey of 31,147 adults which ran for 22 years from 1988 to 2010.

These findings show that people who get 17 to 21 percent of their calories as added sugar have a 38 percent greater risk of death from heart disease compared to persons who get only 8 percent of their calories from added sugar.

And the risk triples for adults who get 25 percent or more of their calories from added sugar.

CALORIES IN SUGAR

A gram of sugar contains four calories. Eight percent of an intake of 2,000 calories a day is 160 calories or 40 grams (160/4). Thus to minimise your risk of heart disease, you need to limit your intake of added sugar to 40 grams a day.

If, instead, you ingest 340 to 420 calories (85 to 105g) a day as added sugar you have a 38 percent higher chance of developing diseases of the heart. And if you take in 500 calories (125g) a day as added sugar you triple your risk.

It's simple really. You can minimise your risk of cardiovascular disease by ensuring that you do not ingest more than 8 percent of you daily calorie requirements from added sugar. For the average person, that's 40g a day of added sugar maximum.

But how can you ensure that the added sugar within your diet does not exceed that maximum?

The simple answer: with great difficulty.

THE SUGAR IN OUR FOOD

Food labelling regulations require the quantity of sugar in a manufactured foodstuff to be shown on the label. So minimising your intake of sugar sounds like a cinch-until you dander down to your local supermarket!

Take cereals for example. A 100g of normal breakfast cereals contains 35g of sugar on average. A reasonably-sized bowl of cereal for breakfast will contain at least 200g, ie 70g of sugar which is well over the 40g limit that minimises your risk of heart disease. And it's still only breakfast time!

Cruise the aisles and read the labels. I have found small tubs of yoghurts that contain 15g of sugar, more than one-third of the daily limit. Sauces, it seems, are loaded with sugar, 44% in the case of a particular sweet chilli sauce.

Next time you are in a supermarket, spend 10 minutes reading labels closely. Then let me know how you can stick to the upper limit of 40g of added sugar a day-without severely restricting your consumption of processed foods.

WHO RECOMMENDATIONS ON SUGAR

For the last ten years, the UN's World Health Organisation has been recommending that a maximum of 10 percent of our daily calories should come from added sugar. For the average adult on 2,000 calories a day, this comes to an upper limit of 50g of added sugar.

The recommended average intake of calories for a child is about 1,200 calories a day. Thus, the WHO's recommended upper limit for a child is 30g a day of added sugar. Go back to the supermarket and check out some more labels.

One can of a sugary drink such as a coke or orangeade exceeds the upper limit of 30g a day for a child, which is not too surprising. But did you know that the sugar in a single-portion tub of yoghurt and a glass of orange juice together can exceed the child's daily limit? Yet compared to a fizzy drink, most of us would, as parents, consider this combination to be a healthier choice.

Throw in beans on toast for tea (7g of sugar) and a jam sandwich (15g plus) along with the yoghurt and orange juice on a regular basis and your kid is well on the road to heart disease in later life.

But even these limits (10 percent of daily calories from added sugar) are now considered too high.

In March 2014, the WHO issued revised recommendations, stating that 5 percent is the more ideal amount of daily calories that should come from added sugar.

This means that, on average, adults should consume no more than 25g of added sugar a day, while children should be limited to 15g a day.

Given the nutritional content of most foodstuffs sold in most supermarkets in the Western world, staying within these limits is almost impossible-unless you give up processed foods entirely.

WHAT TO DO ABOUT ADDED SUGAR IN OUR FOODSTUFFS?

Sugar is added to the stuff we eat by manufacturers and cooks. Then we, the consumers, often add more sugar before we eat. Remember when you used to sprinkle a good spoonful of sugar on your Corn Flakes before adding the full-fat milk?

Reducing the amount of sugar we eat will require drastic changes in how our food is produced and how we consume it.

Manufacturers add sugar (and fat) during processing in order to enhance flavours. This needs to change, even if manufacturers object.

Surely society's ingenious food scientists can come up with tasty foods that do not rely on sugar and fat to be attractive to consumers? Given the right incentives, I'm sure they could.

That incentive can come from legislation forcing them to comply with scientific common sense. The threat of losing a market can be a great incentive for innovation.

In addition, consumers need to learn how to read labels and how to resist being manipulated by advertising. This will require a publicity drive by governments.

Consumers also need to receive advice that is specific. Phrases such as 'sugar needs to be limited' are virtually useless and need to be replaced or expanded with specific recommendations on the maximum amounts people should consume on a daily basis and how to calculate these for food groups.

The good news is that all our tastes and preferences in food (with the exception of mother's milk) are acquired. These tastes can be de-acquired easily enough, as anyone who has switched to a plant-focused diet, like the one I am using to beat my diabetes, will know.

So reducing the added sugars in our food will not present a drastic problem and our taste buds will soon adapt and appreciate the new sensations of taste-provided we know how to assess the sugar in our food.

IMPORTANCE OF ORGANIC DAIRY FOR A HEALTHY LIFESTYLE

Dairy products represent a significant portion of the diets of many people. Diary contains many beneficial vitamins and nutrients, but it is important to get both the right dairy and the right amount of dairy. Otherwise, too much dairy can cause health problems and increase risk for others. When compared to the other food groups, dairy is the one that should always be organic as the differences between conventional and organic dairy are the most significant.

In the United States, recombinant bovine growth hormone, rBGH, is legal and used on most conventional dairy cows because it increases the volume of milk by about 10%. With that increased volume of milk, however, is a greater level of hormones and dairy is the single largest source of ingested hormones with between 60% and 80% of estrogens consumed. In addition to higher level of hormones, conventional milk also contains antibiotics that are given to the cows that are used to treat health problems arising from the hormone injections. Consumption of high levels of estrogens and other hormones can have negative health effects, including increased risk for some cancers. Dairy consumption has been shown to have a major impact on the prevalence of breast cancer As such, it is important to consume organic dairy products, which contain far fewer hormones than conventional dairy products. In addition to organic dairy, dairy products made from skim milk have a significantly lower hormone level than whole-milk varieties because a larger percentage of the hormones are contained in the milk fat.

In addition to consuming only organic dairy, there is a fine line between enough dairy and too much dairy. Because all dairy has estrogens and other hormones, drinking too much dairy, even organic dairy, can cause health issues. Dairy products are extremely high in fat and saturated fat, which are not good for the body in high levels. High fat can make skin oily and increases the amount of mucous production, which can exacerbate congestion and allergies.

Many health benefits come from eating a healthy level of organic dairy products. Dairy contains high levels of Calcium and vitamin D. Calcium has many beneficial effects on the body including maintaining and improving bone strength, keeping blood pressure low, and aiding with weight loss. Vitamin D is also vital in maintaining bone strength. Some specific dairy products have other health benefits including yogurt, which contains enzymes that are aid in digestion and help with overall digestive health. Cottage cheese, on the other hand, is very low fat and contains a lot of protein in addition to calcium.

Diary is an important part of a well-rounded diet, but it is important to consume the right amount of the right type of dairy. Organic dairy contains far fewer hormones and no antibiotics, as opposed to conventional dairy, which greatly reduces many of the long-term health risks associated with dairy consumption. Calcium, protein, vitamin D, and other helpful nutrients are found in dairy products, and they are important in maintaining overall health. By consuming a few servings of organic dairy every day, the body will get the health benefits associated with dairy consumption while minimizing any potential health risks.

30 ALKALINE RECIPES

If you're trying to go alkaline, you'll need to know which foods help your body get to and stay in an alkaline state. The general idea is to eat foods without worrying about an acidic effect, although some are more alkaline than others. It's not necessary to eat only alkaline foods in order to get the body's pH levels to be alkaline, and a certain percentage of foods can and should be acidic, but you should try to choose natural whole foods, like fruits, vegetables and natural grains...

The alkaline diet is one in a string of evidence-based and non-evidence-based diet fads. The idea is to replace acid-forming foods with alkaline foods in order to balance your body's pH levels. Certain food components that can cause acidity in the body include protein, phosphate and sulfur. Alkaline components, on the other hand, include calcium, potassium and magnesium. Acidic foods include meat, poultry, fish, eggs, dairy, alcohol and most grains, while alkaline foods include certain fruits, nuts, legumes and vegetables. There are also foods that are considered neutral, including natural fats, starches and natural sugars.

The alkaline diet is said to improve health and fight serious diseases like cancer. Although the diet is actually quite healthy in essence, there is no evolutionary evidence or human physiological evidence to support some of the many health claims. The reason the diet is a healthy one is because it encourages the consumption of natural unprocessed plant-based foods and lots of fruits and vegetables. But acids, such as amino acids and fatty acids, are actually an extremely important part of any diet in people who don't have an intolerance to them, and should not be cut out.

WHAT SHOULD MY PH LEVELS BE?

This is an important foundation of the alkaline diet, and the ideas behind it. The pH value is a measure of how acidic or alkaline something is, and ranges from 0 to 14. Anything ranging from 0 to 7 is considered acidic, 7 is neutral, and 7 to 14 is alkaline, or basic. However, the pH value in people's bodies varies greatly throughout. Some parts are alkaline and other parts are acidic. The stomach, for example, has hydrochloric acid in it, making it highly acidic, but this is an important digestive necessity in order to break down food. Blood, however, is always slightly alkaline, and it is extremely serious and sometimes fatal if it becomes acidic. Food cannot change your blood pH though, so what you eat has nothing to do with blood becoming acidic. It is only ever caused by a serious disease affecting its level.

HEALTHY ALKALINE FOODS

If you feel that you have an unbalanced diet and eat too many acidic forming foods, like meat, dairy, processed food and alcohol, and not enough alkaline foods, like fruits, vegetables and legumes, then take a look at this list and see if you can increase your alkaline intake…

ALKALINE RECIPE FOR HYDRATING NUTRITIOUS DRINK

1. GO GREEN ALKALINE JUICE

Ingredients

2 Celery Sticks

1/2 Cucumber

1 teaspoon Melrose Organic Barley Grass Powder

1 small piece of Lime, peeled

1/2 ripe Avocado

Ice cubes

How To Prepare This Recipe

Place the ice cubes in a glass.

Juice the celery lime and cucumber and pour over ice to chill the juice

Blend avocado, juice (leave out the ice) and organic barley grass powder until smooth.

serve with a wedge of lime…

You may Drink a la Tequila Style. Lick Celtic Sea Salt, drink and bite the lime!

2. LEMON WATER (AKA SUGAR-FREE LEMON AID)

The most alkaline-forming food you can eat is a lemon. Here is a simple way to get some quick alkalizing going into your body. Lemon juice has great digestive qualities so symptoms of indigestion such as heartburn, bloating and belching are often relieved. Lemons also help cleanse the body of toxins.

Ingredients:

1 lemon

Water

Stevia

Directions:

Wash lemon well

Cut lemon in half, horizontally

Squeeze each half of a lemon

Add to 2 – 4 cups of water. The lemon juice can be diluted more according to taste.

Add stevia to taste.

3. POWER SPINACH SALAD

Greens are the highest alkaline-forming foods and they are full of vitamins A, K, and D. Adding spinach to your meal is an excellent way to alkalize your diet.

This very simple and tasty salad is full of powerfoods. Everyone I have served it to enjoys it very much.

Ingredients:

1 pound fresh spinach

2 tablespoons lemon juice

1/4 cup olive oil

A few drops of stevia

Tamari or Bragg Liquid Aminos to taste

1 avocado, diced

1/4 cup chopped walnuts, roasted until golden

2 mandarin orange sections

Directions:

1. Wash and trim spinach; pat dry with paper towels.

2. Combine lemon juice, oil, stevia and Tamari or Braggs in large bowl; add avocado cubes, coating well with the dressing.

3. Toss spinach and walnuts with avocado and dressing.

4. Add mandarin orange sections and toss spinach salad again.

4. MILLET: THE ALKALIZING GRAIN!

Millet is the only alkalizing grain and it provides many nutrients (15 percent protein), has a sweet nutty flavor and is considered to be one of the most digestible and non-allergenic grains available, and of course it is one of the powerfoods.

It can be a little tasteless. When I first discovered millet 35 years ago, what we did as hippies was to lightly toast it and that has made it a favorite grain of mine!

Ingredients:

1 cup millet

2 1/2 cups water

1/2 tsp. sea salt

Directions:

1. Add millet to a pot with a tight-fitting lid.

2. Dry sauté on medium high heat till golden brown, stirring constantly.

3. Add water and sea salt.

4. Cover with lid, bring to a boil and simmer for 25 to 35 minutes, until all the water is absorbed (millet should be dry).

5. OR (this only works on an electric stove) Cover with lid, bring to a boil and simmer for a few minutes, then turn off the heat.

6. Leave on electric stove burner that you have been cooking on with lid on (do not peek). Leave for 30 minutes; all the water will be absorbed (millet should be dry).

Refreshing Alkaline Recipes to Quench Your Thirst

5. ALKALINE CHLOROPHYLL THRILL

Ingredients

1/2 Lime

1 teaspoon Liquid Chlorophyll

Pure Water

Ice cubes

How To Prepare This Recipe

Place the ice cubes in a tall glass.

Press the lime for its juice and pour over ice together with the chlorophyll.

Add water to fill the glass.

Drink away!

If you like the taste of chlorophyll, add a teaspoon or more into your daily drinking water. It's alkaline and refreshing and different from the sodium bicarbonate taste!

6. BUCKWHEAT CREPES WITH ALKALINE SYRUP

Ingredients

1 cup Buckwheat flour

2 Eggs *

1 tablespoon Olive Oil

1/2 teaspoon Celtic Sea Salt

1/2 litre Water

3 tablespoons Olive Oil

For a less rich slice use fresh tomatoes

*1 egg = 1 tablespoon ground flax seed simmered in 3 tablespoons of water

How To Prepare This Recipe

In the mixer, add all ingredients for 1 minute.

If no mixer, put flour in a bowl add oil the eggs and celtic salt. Mix vigorously.

Slowly add the water.

Mix quickly for 3 minutes to obtain a smooth mixture.

Let it stand for 2 hours, with a cloth over the top of the bowl. Oil your pan and flip both sides of your crepes when the pan is hot.

7. BUTTERNUT PUMPKIN ALKALINE SOUP

Ingredients

2 Butternut Squash

1 Onion

3-4 cups Water with Celtic Sea Salt

1 can Coconut Milk

Cinnamon and Nutmeg

How To Prepare This Recipe

Cut squash in half and remove seeds remove skin and cut flesh in small pieces.

Cut onion in small pieces.

Bring water to boil with the salt and add veggies and cinnamon and nutmeg.

When all veggies soft…blend with the mixer.

Serve in bowl and onion rings to garnish.

8. ALKALINE CHAR GRILLED CALAMARI

Ingredients

2 Calamari

Garlic mayo to taste

4 cups Rocket leaves

2 tablespoons Balsamic Vinegar

2 tablespoons Flax Seed Oil

3 tablespoons Lemon Grass

2 Garlic cloves, minced

Celtic Salt

1 cup Spelt Bread Crumbs

3 tablespoons Olive Oil

How To Prepare This Recipe

Slice your calamari and dip it in a mix of bread crumbs, garlic and lemon grass.

Put your olive oil in a pan and heat up gently. Fry the calamari for 3 minutes and add 1/4 cup water, cover and simmer until calamari are tender.

In a bowl mix rocket, flax oil and vinegar, add salt to taste.

Mix calamari into the bowl and add rest of the cubs mix too.

8.1. CHICKPEA AND SPINACH CURRY

Servings: 6 Preparation time: 10 minutes

Ingredients:

1 cup coarsely chopped onion

1-1/2 Tbsp fresh ginger, chopped or grated

1 tsp olive oil or virgin coconut oil

1-1/2 tsp red curry powder

1 19 oz can chickpeas, rinsed and drained

1 14 oz can diced tomatoes with liquid

1 10 oz bag spinach

1/2 cup water

1/4 tsp salt (optional)

Directions:

Put the ginger and onion in a food blender/mixer until it is minced.

Heat oil gently in large skillet over medium high heat.

Add onion mixture and curry. Sauté 3 minutes.

Add chickpeas and tomatoes; simmer for 2 minutes.

Stir in spinach, water and salt.

Cook another minute or until spinach wilts.

9. AVOCADO FRUIT SALAD NUMBER OF SERVING: 8 PREPARATION TIME: 10 MINUTES

Ingredients:

1/2 ripe avocado, seeded and peeled (1/2 sliced into 8 portions, 1/2" cubed)

1-1/2 Tbsp olive oil

2 Tbsp raspberry vinegar

1 tsp grated lime peel

1 Tbsp fresh lime juice

1 Tbsp fresh chopped basil leaves

1/2 tsp dry mustard

1/4 tsp salt

1/4 tsp pepper

1 10 oz package mixed baby greens

4 kiwi, peeled and sliced in half rounds

4 grapefruit

2 cups sliced strawberries

2 star fruits, sliced

Directions:

Salad Dressing - In a small bowl, whisk together remaining ingredients, set aside.

Salad - In a large salad bowl, combine baby greens, kiwi, grapefruit, strawberries and star fruit.

Pour on dressing and toss to coat.

Top with avocado slices.

10. VERY VEGGIE SALAD

Number of Servings: 4 Preparation time: 15 minutes

Ingredients:

4 cups raw spinach

4 cups romaine lettuce

2 cups chopped red, yellow, orange bell pepper

2 cups cherry tomatoes

1 cup chopped broccoli

1 cup chopped cauliflower

1 cup sliced yellow squash

1 cup sliced zucchini

2 cups sliced cucumber

2 cups chopped baby carrots

Directions:

Wash all of the vegetables and mix them together in a large mixing bowl.

Top this colorful meal with a nonfat or low-fat dressing of your choice

11. SOUP OF FRESH GARDEN VEGETABLES

You need a small zucchini, some carrots, a celery stalk, two teaspoonfuls salt, a teaspoon fresh basil, three asparagus stalks, broccoli, five teaspoonfuls yeast-free vegetable broth and a yellow onion.

First boil the broth and onion in a pot of water and then chop and shred carrots, zucchini, broccoli, asparagus and celery stalk in a food processor. As vegetables should be tender and not boiled for these diet recipes, add vegetables only after turning off the cooker and leave to tenderize. Mix all the boiled ingredients in a blender till thick while adding some salt to taste.

12. AVOCADO FRUIT SALAD

You need half an avocado which is seeded and peeled into 8 ½" cubes, 2 tbsp raspberry vinegar, a tbsp each of fresh lime juice and chopped basil leaves, 1 ½ tbsp olive oil, 1 tsp grated lime peel, ½ tsp dry mustard, ¼ tsp each of salt and pepper, 4 kiwi peeled and sliced in half rounds, 10 oz pack mixed baby greens, 4 grapefruit and 2 cups each of sliced star fruits and strawberries.

First combine grapefruit, strawberries, kiwi, baby greens and star fruit in a salad bowl. Then make a salad dressing in a small bowl by whisking remaining ingredients. Pour the dressing on the salad and top with avocado slices.

13. FRESH VEGGIE SALAD

You need 4 cups each of raw spinach and romaine lettuce, 2 cups each of cherry tomatoes, sliced cucumber, chopped baby carrots and chopped red, orange and yellow bell pepper and a cup each of chopped broccoli, sliced yellow squash, zucchini and cauliflower.

Just wash all these vegetables. Mix in a large mixing bowl and top off with a non-fat or low-fat dressing of your choice.

Our bodies are similar to pools in two ways: pools and humans are both bodies of water (pun very much intended), and we both have a pH level that needs to be monitored and maintained. pH stands for power of Hydrogen and shows the levels of Hydrogen ions in a given body .

The human body wants to be balanced, and for us a balanced pH level is slightly alkaline. The scale ranges from 0 – 14, the lower end of the scale is acidic, leaving the higher end to be alkaline. The perfect spot for our bodies is 7.30-7.45. How do we incorporate alkalines into our diets?

We Don't Need Chlorine

An alkaline-diet helps you get up and go in the morning. It boosts your energy without a crash, and you feel more naturally awake in the morning. It's also nearly impossible to lose weight if your body is over-acidic, which most of us are.

So I've compiled this comprehensive list of alkaline soups, salads, sides, snacks, and meals.

SOUPS

Alkaline Carrot and Mushroom Soup

Mushrooms help neutralize stomach acids and carrots are a great source of B-vitamins, and other minerals like calcium, iron, and magnesium. Plus with a wonderful colour, texture, and taste, how could you say no to this soup?

14. CHILLED AVOCADO AND TOMATO SOUP

A perfect summer soup. Avocados are the food most typically associated with an alkaline diet. They are rich in potassium which regulates blood pressure, and the fatty-acids lower your cholesterol.

15. RAW AVOCADO-BROCCOLI SOUP WITH CHESTNUTS

All dark leafy greens are high on the alkaline scale, and broccoli is no exception. Mixed with avocado, you've got a soup that is high in alkaline-forming properties, and high is amazing-taste as well.

SALADS

16. AVOCADO SALAD WITH WILD GARLIC

You'll notice that avocado shows up in most of these recipes. Wild garlic is also a huge health-booster with more minerals than regular garlic, it is the healthiest choice for salads.

17. FRESH GARDEN VEGETABLE SALAD

Always go fresh – fresh veggies for your salad, fresh herbs and cold-pressed oils for dressings will keep you feeling fresh all day long.

18. CHINESE-STYLE CUCUMBER SALAD

Cucumber, garlic, and sesame seed oil – that's it here. Super easy, super alkaline, this simple salad is a great start to your alkaline dinner.

19. ALKALINE MEDITERRANEAN SALAD

A mediterranean diet is one of the best. All fresh veggies help you live a happier, more holistic lifestyle.

SNACKS AND SIDES

20. MEDITERRANEAN BELL PEPPERS

Low in calories, high in vitamin C, folic acid, and beta carotene, bell peppers are a great alkaline food. Again, the mediterranean diet wins.

21. MASHED BRUSSELS SPROUTS WITH CAULIFLOWER

Brussels sprouts are super-high in alkaline salts and minerals like phosphorus, magnesium, potassium, and other minerals including iron. This side is good for the whole family!

22. AVOCADO-TOMATO-SALSA WITH POTATOES

A popular appetizer with guests, you can also serve it without the potatoes as a dip.

23. ALKALINE POTATO SALAD

Every ingredient in this will help balance your pH levels and fill you up! A great ease-in to the alkaline diet.

MAINS

24. QUINOA PASTA WITH TOMATO ARTICHOKE SAUCE

An alkaline diet doesn't mean you need to give up pasta. Just remember to use quinoa or spelt pasta, always use lots of fresh veggies, and leave out the red meat.

25. ALKALINE VEGGIE STIR-FRY WITH LEEKS AND KOHLRABI

The original recipe is from a family in Switzerland, and contains interesting herbs and rich alkaline veggies. Try it today, and let us know how it goes!

26. ALKALINE RATATOUILLE

Traditionally a stewed French dish, this ratatouille is all alkaline forming, so dig in and bon apetit.

27. POTATO PUMPKIN PATTIES

Pumpkins are high in alkaline forming properties and low in calories, which makes them a perfect potato patty pair.

28. SPICY TOMATO SHAKE

Sounds weird, tastes great. Low in calories and totally alkaline, cucumbers are also great helps to your kidneys, bladder, and liver.

29. ALKALINE VEGGIE POWER SMOOTHIE

This anytime snack gives energizes you any time of the day: breakfast, lunch, dinner, or beyond! Stay smooth with this Power Smoothie

30. GREEN POWER COCKTAIL

Green shakes and smoothies are always jam-packed with vitamins, nutrients, and alkaline-forming foods. Give this drink a try when you need a power boost.

CONCLUSION

It can be helpful to refer to a list of specific foods, but generally you should attempt to eat an abundance of fresh fruits and vegetables every day. Salads are always a good choice. Make sure to drink lots of water, vegetable juice, or herbal teas. Avoid processed foods, fried foods, chocolates, foods that contain added sugars, and junk foods. Instead of adding sugar or salt to the foods you cook, try using healthy and flavorful herbs and spices. Last but not least, keep in mind that if you overcook your foods, you will be losing much of the nutritional value.

Oranges and lemons known for being acidic convert into alkaline after digestion and absorbed by the body is a good alkaline diet. Generally, we must consume 75% of alkaline food daily. The higher the amount of alkaline foods we put into our system, the greater the neutralization of the acidic condition in our body.

A healthy and balanced diet is more alkaline than acid. Based upon your blood type, the diet should be made up of 60 to 80% alkaline foods and 20 to 40% acidic foods. Normally, the A and AB blood types require the most alkaline diet while the O and B blood types require more animal products in their diet. But keep in mind; if you're in pain, you're acidic.

Transitioning to an alkaline diet requires a shift in one's attitude about food. It is helpful to explore new tastes and textures while making small changes and improving old habits